MAXIMIZING MOBILITY AFTER STROKE
Nursing the Acute Patient

George I. Turnbull and Patricia A. Bell

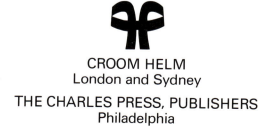

CROOM HELM
London and Sydney

THE CHARLES PRESS, PUBLISHERS
Philadelphia

British Library Cataloguing in Publication Data

Turnbull, George I.
    Maximizing mobility after stroke: nursing
    the acute patient.
    1. Cerebrovascular disease – Treatment
    I. Title   II. Bell, Patricia A.
    616.8'1   RC338.5
    ISBN 0-7099-2493-3   ✓ B

The Charles Press, Publishers,
Suite 14K, 1420 Locust Street,
Philadelphia,
Pennsylvania 19102

ISBN 0-914783-10-6

Library of Congress Number: 85-071509

Printed and bound in Great Britain

The preparation of this handbook was made possible by a grant
from the Nova Scotia Heart Foundation.

MAXIMIZING MOBILITY AFTER STROKE

L

Kil
Co
01-

This
stan
it ma
for r

3/88

12/8

7/8

Table of Contents

Aims and Objectives 3
The Stroke Problem 4
Rehabilitation Considerations 4
Current Principles of Rehabilitation 5
Arrangement of the Patient's Room 7
Visitors 9
Approaching the Patient 11
Positioning the Patient in Bed 13
    supine 13
    side lying on the sound side 14
    side lying on the affected side 15
    long sitting 16
Moving the Patient in Bed 18
    supine to side lying on the affected side 18
    supine to side lying on the sound side 20
    side lying to supine 21
    bridging (bed pan routine) 22
    moving the patient in bed 23
    side lying to sitting over the edge of the bed 24
Seating Requirements 28
    chairs 28
    wheelchairs 30
    wheelchair accessories 31
Positioning the Patient in a Chair 32
Positioning the Patient in a Wheelchair 34
Repositioning the Patient in the Chair or Wheelchair .. 36
    independently 36
    with assistance 38
Propelling the Wheelchair 40
Transfers 42
    edge of the bed to the chair 42
    chair to wheelchair 42
    wheelchair to toilet 50
    toilet to wheelchair 51
    chair or wheelchair to standing (two operators) ... 52
    chair or wheelchair to standing (one operator) 54
    chair or wheelchair to standing (independently) ... 56
Activities in Standing 58
    position and support of the operators 58
    correct hand hold when standing 59
Walking the Patient 60
Range of Motion Exercises 62
    general guidelines 62
    upper limb 62
    lower limb 66

Activities of Daily Living (A.D.L.) 68
    general guidelines 68
Conclusion 70
Selected Glossary 71
Suggested Further Reading 73

2

Aims and Objectives

The writing of this book has been prompted by the firm belief that the acute-care management of the stroke patient significantly influences the eventual functional outcome. The book is designed to be used as a working reference for nursing and physiotherapy staff and to promote a coordination of effort to the maximum benefit of the patient.

With this in mind, the aims and objectives of this publication are as follows:

1. To communicate contemporary functional re-education philosophies pertaining to the management of the acute stroke patient.

2. To apply these techniques to common nursing procedures.

3. To assist in coordinating the management of the acute stroke patient between nursing staff and physiotherapists.

4. To maximize the short and long term functional recovery of the stroke patient by the coordinated application of remedial procedures.

The format of this book has been arranged to promote the attainment of its objectives. Each application is described under the heading " Procedure" with the rationale explained in the "Reason" category. Where attention to specific points is indicated a "Note" section is included. The text of this book has deliberately been kept to a minimum to promote its quick reference function. Similarly, terminology has been kept constant throughout to avoid confusion and a degree of repetition has also been used to emphasise important points. A selected glossary explaining terms commonly used by physiotherapists has been included.

It is the hope of the authors that this book will be used extensively as a working document to the benefit of all stroke patients.

The Stroke Problem

Cerebrovascular accident (CVA) or stroke, is a focal neurological disorder with an abrupt onset and rapid development. The resultant central nervous system damage is caused by interruption of the blood supply in the vascular network of the brain and may have either an ischaemic or haemorrhagic basis. The patient experiences a variety of symptoms one of which may be a loss of motor function on the opposite side of the body to the involved cerebral hemisphere (hemiplegia). This may be complicated by other disturbances such as alterations of sensation, perception, vision and speech.

It has been estimated that there are 500,000 new strokes each year in the United States of which 300,000 survive. Of the survivors the majority suffer neurological dysfunction and physical disability of varying degrees and it has been shown that stroke is the third leading cause of death and the greatest cause of long term disability in the United States.

In Canada, it has been reported that each year, one of every five hundred people suffers stroke resulting in 40,000 new cases per annum.

One of the principal considerations in the management of stroke is the functional rehabilitation process which is undertaken as soon as the medical condition of the patient becomes stable.

Rehabilitation Considerations

In the past, rehabilitation procedures were designed to teach the patient to compensate for their disability by emphasizing treatment of the sound non-involved side of the body. A greater understanding of neurophysiological processes has, more recently, led to current methods which promote functional re-education of the hemiplegic side **(affected side)**. It is the purpose of this book to apply this contemporary philosophy to common nursing procedures required in the management of stroke in the acute hospital setting.

Rehabilitation efforts are maximized when they are initiated **as early as possible**. During the acute phase it is important that strategies which will complement later rehabilitation efforts are implemented. To this end, control of abnormal patterns of spasticity and encouragement of normal movement are of prime importance.

A major role in the care of the stroke patient is played by the nurse. Although the patient will spend time with the physiotherapist and other health care workers, the majority of time is spent on the ward where most of the care is provided by the nursing staff. It is therefore of considerable importance that the nurse is well acquainted with current stroke rehabilitation concepts and procedures. This will ensure a consistent and coordinated team approach to the management of stroke in the acute setting which will complement future functional recovery of the patient.

Current Principles of Rehabilitation

The following basic goals and principles form the foundation for the total management process in the overall rehabilitation effort.

Prevention of Complications

The risks associated with immobility and loss of normal motor function are of major concern in the management of acute stroke. Preventive passive and active range of motion exercises have been designed to meet the specific needs of the stroke patient. Frequent turnings, combined with the application of recommended positions of bedrest will help prevent the formation of decubitii and will inhibit the development of spasticity.

The role of the nurse is of prime importance in these aspects of the care of the patient.

Inhibition of Spasticity

Spasticity (abnormal increases in muscle tone) interferes with the ability of the patient to move normally. Spasticity develops insidiously a few days after the stroke has occurred and gradually replaces the initial complete paralysis of the muscles of the **affected side** of the body. The prevention of the development of spasticity can be achieved through careful positioning of the patient **at all times**. It is of great importance to prevent spasticity and abnormal primitive reflexes in order to ensure that the likelihood of normal functional movement being regained is maximized.

Reeducation of the Affected Side

The objective of current functional rehabilitation is the reeducation of the **affected side** to its fullest potential. The patient must continually be encouraged to use the **affected limbs** in a functional manner throughout all daily activities. The concept of symmetry of the body and limbs is an integral part of this reeducation process. Symmetry occurs when both halves of the body contribute to the achievement of functional activity by working together in a coor-

5

dinated manner. The person who has suffered a stroke is asymmetrical initially. A concentrated and coordinated effort must be made to encourage the patient to use the **affected limbs** as much and as normally as possible thus encouraging and promoting symmetry.

Independence

Maximum functional independence of the patient is the ultimate goal of coordinated rehabilitation efforts. This principle must be kept in mind by all who are involved in the care of the patient particularly nursing and physiotherapy staff.

Every attempt should be made to encourage independence while adhering to the general principles outlined in this book.

Arrangement of the Patient's Room

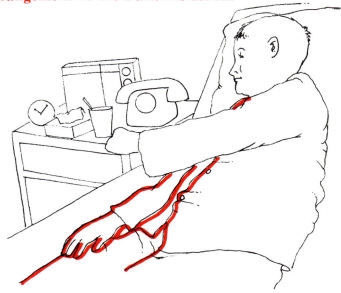

Procedure

- position bedside lockers, tables, pictures and other sources of interest to the **affected side** of the patient.

Reasons

- minimizes any tendency by the patient to ignore the **affected side.**
- stimulates the patient to the environment on the **affected side.**
- encourages the patient to look and reach towards the **affected side.**
- promotes weight bearing through the **affected hip.**
- reduces abnormal muscle tone by rotation of the spine.

Note

- the procedure described above is consistent with current rehabilitation approaches and will complement their effectiveness.

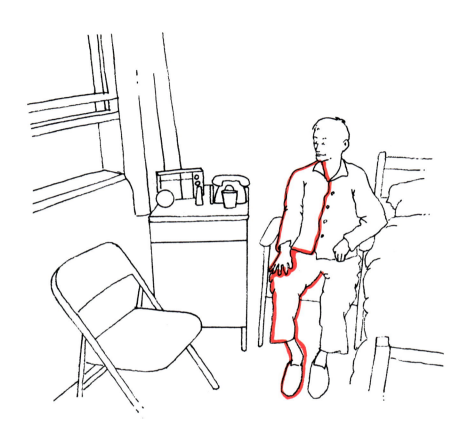

Visitors

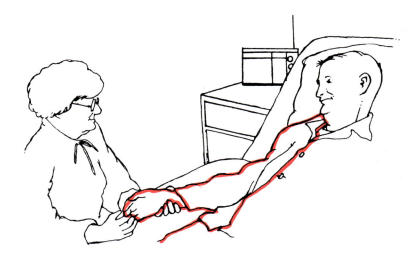

- all seating arrangements for visitors should be placed to the **affected** side of the patient.

Reasons

- minimizes any tendency by the patient to ignore the **affected side**.
- encourages patient to look towards the **affected side**.
- introduces family members at an early stage to approaching patient on the **affected side**.

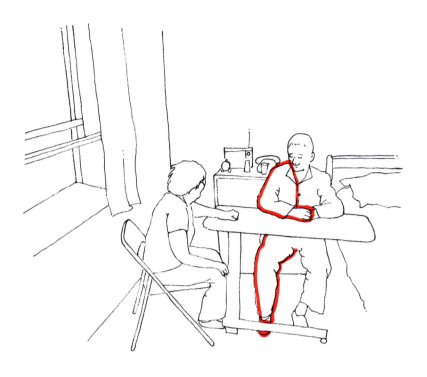

Note

- close family members should be encouraged to touch and rub the **affected hand** of the patient to provide sensory stimulation. This may reduce apprehensions in the minds of relatives towards the condition of the patient while allowing them to feel part of the rehabilitation process.

Approaching the Patient

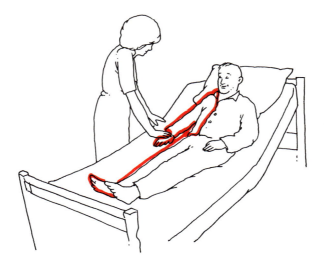

Procedure

- nursing care should be administered when possible from the **affected side** of the patient.

Reasons

- minimizes any tendency by the patient to ignore the **affected side**.
- encourages the patient to look towards the **affected side**.
- prevents the patient from compensating for the paralysis with the sound side which is **unacceptable** and which will interefere with rehabilitation.

Note

- when a visual field deficit is present this regime should still be applied. The patient, with encouragement, will learn to compensate for the deficit by turning his head.
- **do not** nurse patient from the sound side unless absolutely essential.

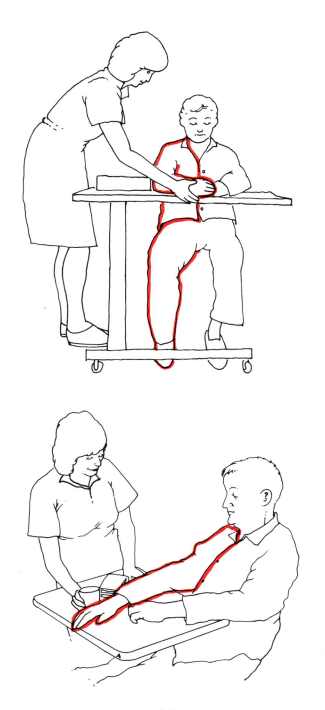

Positioning the Patient in Bed

Supine (Lying on back)

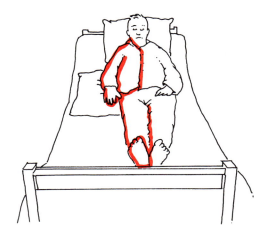

Procedure

- the patient's head is straight and in the midposition.
- on the **affected side**: Place pillows under the shoulder girdle region and arm, hip and knee. Keep the hand flat with the fingers extended.
  Ensure that the legs are resting in a neutral position and are not excessively externally rotated.

Reasons

- proper body alignment encourages a normal body image.
- pillows placed under the **affected arm** aids in the prevention and reduction of oedema.
- pillows are placed behind the shoulder to prevent trauma (subluxation) to the shoulder joint from lack of muscle tone and also to reduce spasticity.
- a pillow behind the hip will aid in the prevention of the development of spasticity.

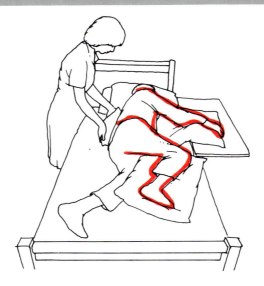

Procedure

- the **affected shoulder** must be placed well forward.
- keep the **affected arm** outstretched.
- a pillow can be placed behind the back for added support.
- the legs are best kept flexed at the hip and knee joints with the **affected knee** foremost and a pillow between the legs.

Reasons

- the above position allows the patient to be comfortable while preventing the development of spasticity.
- stimulates normal sensation on the **affected side**.

Side Lying on the Affected Side

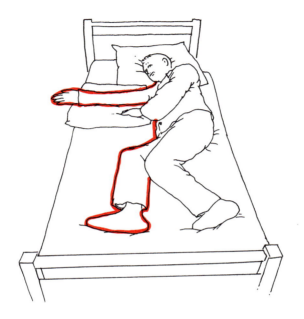

Procedure

- place a pillow under the **affected outstretched arm**.

Reasons

- this position allows the patient to be comfortable with the simultaneous inhibition of abnormal motor patterns which will interfere with future functional rehabilitation efforts.

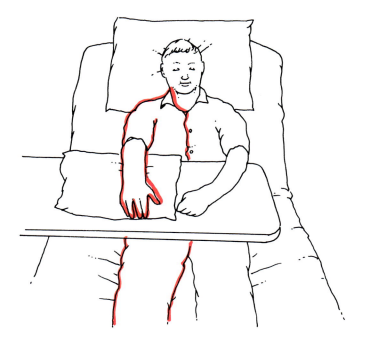

- the head of the patient is situated in the midposition.
- place a pillow under the **affected arm,** keeping the hand flat and palm downwards.
- the patient must be placed in a symmetrical position.

Reasons

- this position allows the patient to be comfortable with simultaneous control of spasticity.

Note

- it may be necessary for support to be placed on the lateral aspect of the **affected leg** as there is a tendency for this leg to externally rotate and thus interfere with normal body alignment.

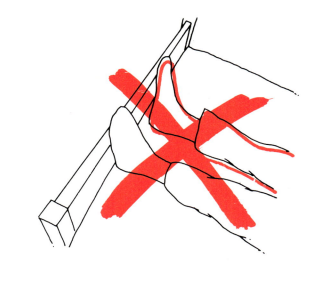

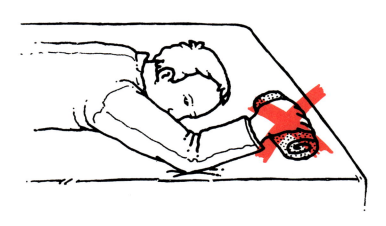

Note

- **footboards** and **handrolls** must **not** be used as they tend to stimulate an increase in spasticity even when the limb appears flaccid.

Moving the Patient in Bed

Supine to Side Lying on the Affected Side (Rolling)

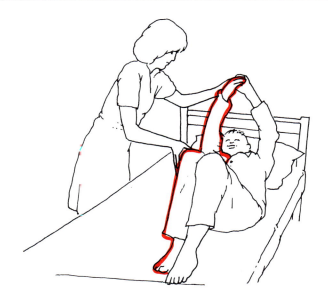

Procedure

- have the patient bend the knees with feet flat on the bed and clasp his hands together interlacing the fingers.

Reasons

- promotes symmetrical movement of the limbs.
- encourages the use of the **affected side** of the patient.
- promotes sensory stimulation of the **affected hand**.

Note

- provide assistance only when necessary.
- the nurse may have to stabilise the affected foot.

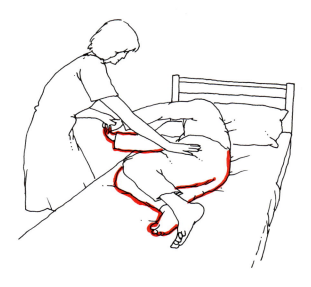

Procedure

- the patient reaches upwards with the arms, hands towards the ceiling.
- utilizing both arms and legs the patient rolls to the **affected side**.

Reasons

- promotes symmetrical movement of the limbs.
- encourages the use of the **affected side** of the patient.
- minimizes the possibility of the **affected side** being "forgotten" with an increased possibility of damage to the shoulder joint.

Note

- it is **unacceptable** for the patient to grasp handrails or bedsheets when rolling. This discourages the use of the **affected side** and may stimulate unwanted patterns of spasticity which will interfere with the re-education of normal functional movement.
- when the patient has rolled to the desired position ensure that the correct positioning procedure is followed (see page 16).

19

Moving the Patient in Bed (cont.)

Supine to Side Lying on the Sound Side (Rolling)

Procedure

- the procedure for rolling towards the non affected side is identical to the method described for rolling on to the **affected side**.

Reason

- further promotes symmetrical movement of the limbs.
- encourages use of the **affected side** of the patient.
- minimizes the likelihood of damage to the **affected shoulder**.

Note

- provide assistance only when necessary.
- when the patient has rolled to the desired position ensure that the correct positioning procedure is followed (see page 15).

Side Lying to Supine

Procedure

- have the patient interlace his fingers and bend both knees keeping his feet together.
- utilizing both arms and legs the patient rolls on to his back while attempting to keep the knees bent and the feet together.

Reasons

- encourages the use of the **affected side** of the body.
- promotes symmetrical movement of the limbs.

Note

- provide assistance only when necessary.
- the nurse should stabilize both of the patient's feet so that the knees are maintained in flexion and the feet remain in contact with the bed (upon completion of the procedure, the whole sole of both feet must be firmly in contact with the bed).

Camden P.L.

Moving the Patient in Bed (cont.)

Bridging (Bed Pan Routine)

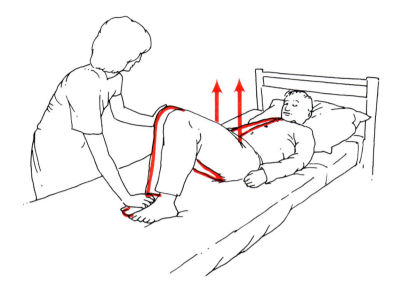

Procedure

- have the patient bend the knees up and raise the hips off the bed pressing **both** feet into the bed.

Reasons

- promotes symmetrical movement of the limbs.
- permits weight bearing through the **affected foot**.
- encourages the use of the **affected side** of the patient.

Note

- provide assistance only when necessary.
- sometimes it is necessary to stabilize the feet of the patient and provide support at the knees.

Moving the Patient in Bed

Procedure

- the patient bends both knees up so that the soles of his feet are firmly in contact with the bed.
- the nurses link hands under the patient's back and ask the patient to push with his feet.
- as the patient pushes, the nurses guide him up towards the top of the bed.

Reasons

- allows the patient to use his **affected leg**.
- the patient contributes to the procedure thus encouraging independence.

Note

- encourage the patient to push with both legs as much as possible.
- be particularly careful to avoid pulling on the **affected shoulder joint**.

Moving the Patient in Bed (cont.)

Side Lying to Sitting Over the Edge of the Bed

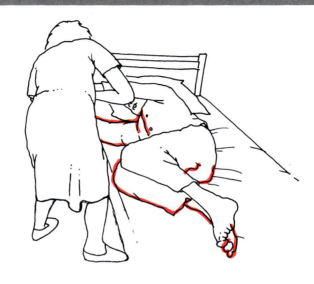

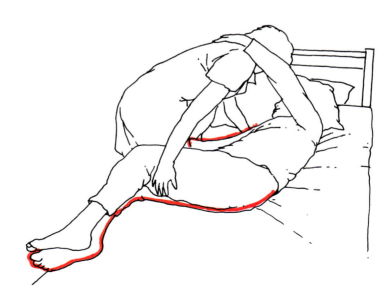

- the starting position is side lying on the **affected side** with both knees slightly flexed.

Reasons

- allows the patient to use the **affected side** when moving.

Procedure

- the operator places one supporting arm under the patient's axilla and supports the patient's trunk with the same hand.
- the other hand of the operator is placed under both knees of the patient.
- the patient may place the non-affected arm around the neck of the operator.

Reasons

- allows the nurse maximum control over the trunk while protecting the **affected shoulder joint** of the patient.

Moving the Patient in Bed (cont.)

Side Lying to Sitting Over the Edge of the Bed (cont.)

Procedure

- the nurse pivots the patient into the sitting position by lifting the patient under the trunk and guiding the legs over the edge of the bed.
- the patient **should** be encouraged to assist as much as possible.

Reasons

- encourages the use of the **affected side** of the patient.

Note

- care must be taken not to allow the patient to pull excessively with the sound arm as this will result in increased spasticity and possible injury to the operator.

Procedure

- raise the patient to sitting over the side of the bed.
- ensure that the feet of the patient are placed on a flat surface. If the feet do not reach the floor so that the whole of both soles are firmly on the ground then a small footstool should be used.

Reasons

- a firm surface under the feet promotes weight bearing through the legs and encourages symmetry of the lower limbs.
- stimulation of only the ball of the foot will result in increased spasticity of the **affected lower limbs**.

Note

- assistance in bringing the legs over the side of the bed may often be necessary in the early stages.
- when the patient wishes to go back to bed, the same procedure is followed but in reverse order.

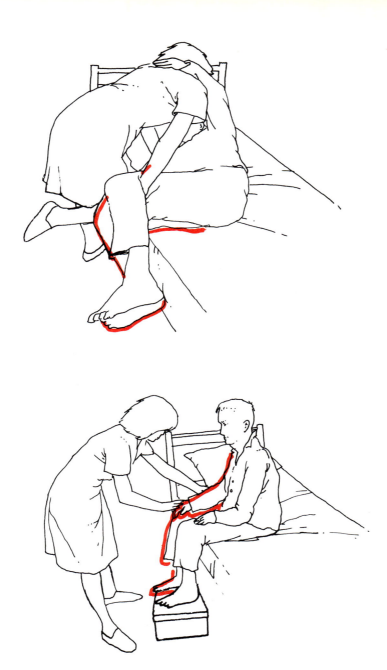

Seating Requirements

Chairs

Ideal Chair

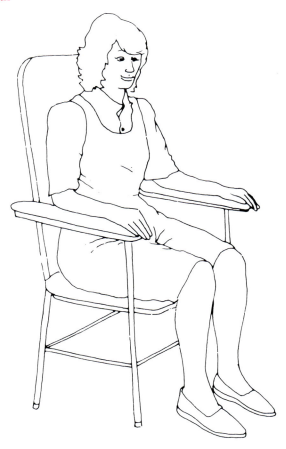

- firm, level seat.
- arm rests.
- upright back with proper support.
- appropriate height (feet should rest flat on the floor).
- weight of the patient is mostly on the hips and feet and is equal on both sides of the body.
- the patient should be able to carry out some independent adjustments of position when seated in this chair.

Unsuitable Chair

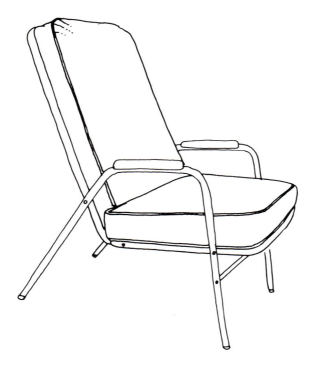

- seat is too low (independent sitting and rising from the chair is very difficult).
- concentration of the weight is against the back of the patient.
- the patient **cannot** carry out independent adjustments from this position.

Wheelchairs

Ideal Wheelchair

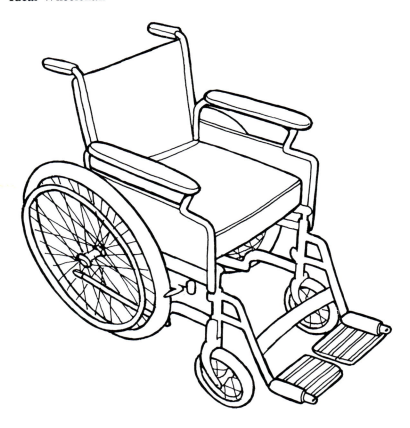

- comfortable, firm seat.
- good supporting back rest.
- swing away footrests.
- footrests at the appropriate height (knees at 90 degrees).
- removable arm rests.

Arm gutters

- arm gutters tend to put the **affected upper limb** in a nonfunctional position and out of sight of the patient. The patient is less likely to acknowledge the limb under these circumstances. Their application, therefore, is **not** recommended.

Table Attachments

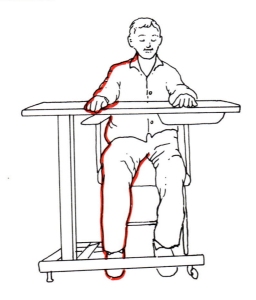

- a bedside table can be used when table attachments are not acessible for the following reasons:
  a) both hands can be placed in the visual field of the patient.
  b) functional use of the **affected side** is promoted.
  c) encourages weight bearing through the **affected elbow and shoulder** which may substantially reduce the occurrance of pain in the shoulder.

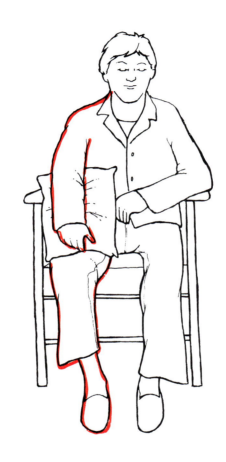

- ensure head is in the midline position.
- equal weight bearing through both hips.
- hips, knees and ankles are at right angles to each other.
- both feet are flat on the floor (six to eight inches apart).
- shoulders and arms properly supported on either a pillow or a table.
- **affected hand** is flat with fingers extended.

Reasons

- promotes normal body alignment.
- allows maximum comfort of the patient with a simultaneous control of spasticity.
- permits equal distribution of weight through both hips and both feet.
- encourages an appreciation of normal sensation.
- encourages the relearning of sitting balance.

Procedure

- position bedside lockers, tables, pictures and other sources of interest on the **affected side** of the patient.

Reasons

- minimizes any tendency by the patient to ignore the **affected side**.
- encourages the patient to look and reach towards the **affected hip**.
- reduces abnormal muscle tone by rotating the spine.

Positioning the Patient in a Wheelchair

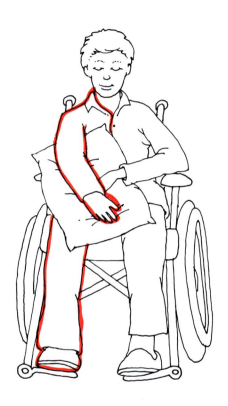

- ensure head is in the midline position.
- equal weight bearing through both hips.
- hip, knee and ankle joints are at right angles.
- feet flat on the footrests.
- **affected arm and shoulder** properly supported on either a pillow or table.
- **affected hand** is flat with the fingers extended.

Reasons

- promotes good body alignment.
- ensures the comfort of the patient with a subsequent reduction in abnormal muscle tone.
- prevents abnormal patterns of spasticity.
- supports the **affected shoulder joint**.
- encourages symmetrical equal weight through both upper limbs.

Note

- the symmetrical position of the body is designed to encourage equal use of both limbs and promotes a normal appreciation of body image.

Repositioning the Patient in the Chair or Wheelchair

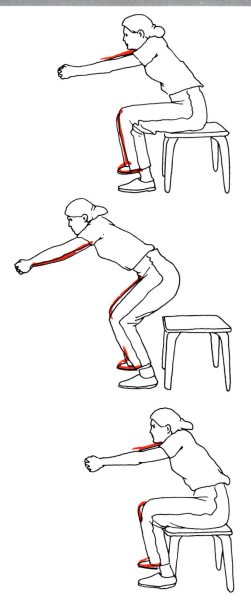

- the patient clasps hands together.
- the feet of the patient are flat on the floor and slightly under the patient.
- the patient reaches forward with the arms raising the hips off the chair.
- return to symmetrical sitting position.

Reasons

- promotes symmetrical movement of the limbs.
- encourages the use of the **affected side**.
- permits equal weight bearing through both feet.

Note

- this fairly advanced procedure may not be attainable in some patients in the early stages however it should be encouraged if at all possible.

Repositioning the Patient in the Chair or Wheelchair (Cont.)

With assistance

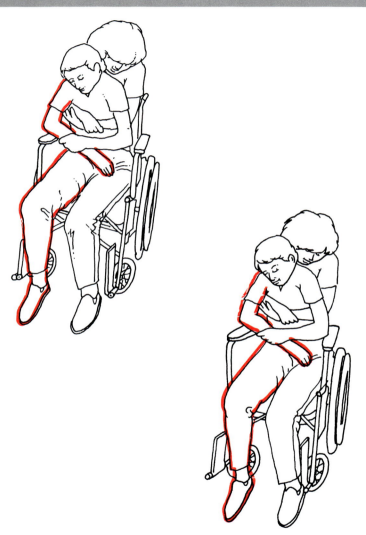

Procedure

- position the feet of the patient flat on the floor.
- the operator stands behind the wheelchair.
- hold the patient around the chest beneath the arms.
- the patient holds the **affected arm** against the body with the sound arm.
- lift the patient back into the chair and reposition symmetrically.

Reasons

- allows the patient to be repositioned safely with minimal effort by the operator.
- prevents any trauma to the **affected shoulder joint**.

Note

- encourage the patient to assist with this procedure by pressing both feet on to the floor.
- employ proper back mechanics when lifting the patient (lift with the legs).
- care must be taken to avoid pulling on the affected shoulder joint.

Propelling the Wheelchair

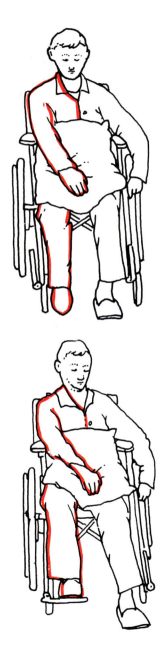

Procedure

- the chair is generally propelled by the sound limbs of the patient.
- the chair is directed by the sound foot using a heel-toe pattern (the same as that used in the support phase of normal walking).

Reasons

- permits the patient greater independence.

Note

- the use of the **affected limbs** are employed as soon as possible, particularly the lower limb. This procedure encourages the use of the **affected leg** and assists in the relearning of a normal, safe and symmetrical walking pattern.

Procedure

- secure the brakes with the sound hand and, when possible, the **affected hand**.

Reasons

- reaching across the **affected side** to the brake promotes a reduction in spasticity by the rotation of the spine.
- promotes weight bearing through the **affected hip**.
- promotes safe functional wheelchair independence.

Sitting on the Edge of the Bed to the Chair

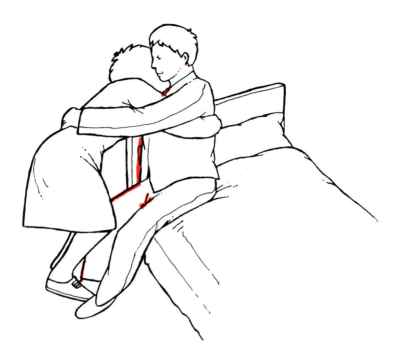

Procedure

- the chair is placed next to the bed on the **affected side** of the patient.

Reasons

- permits the patient to transfer **towards** the **affected side**.
- increases the awareness and encourages the use of the **affected side**.

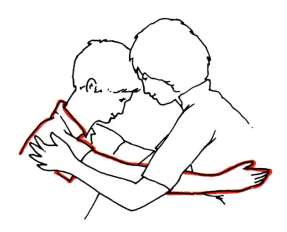

Procedure

- the operator places a supporting hand on the **affected scapula** with the arm of the patient well supported.
- the **affected knee** is braced on either side.

Reasons

- provides support and stability for the patient where it is required most.
- protects the shoulder joint from potential injury.
- encourages equal weight bearing through both lower limbs.

Note

- the balance mechanisms that are encouraged in the **affected leg** when transferring will assist later in the rehabilitation of a normal walking pattern.

Sitting on the Edge of the Bed to the Chair (cont.)

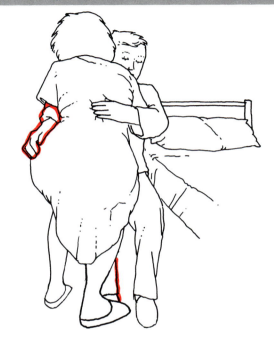

Procedure

- the patient brings the hips to the edge of the bed with feet flat on the floor.
- leans forward to raise the hips off the bed.
- it is only necessary to **stand part ways**.

Reasons

- ensures equal weight bearing through both feet.
- standing part ways requires less assistance from the operator than erect standing.

- pivot the patient to the carefully positioned chair.
- the patient leans forward and bends both knees when sitting.

Reasons

- pivoting is easily performed with minimal energy expenditure.
- encourages the participation of the patient independently with support from the nurse.

Note

- the above procedure is easily performed by one operator.
- with two people, the second operator is positioned between the bed and the chair and will guide the hips of the patient.
- when the patient sits down again on the bed the same procedure is followed but in reverse order.

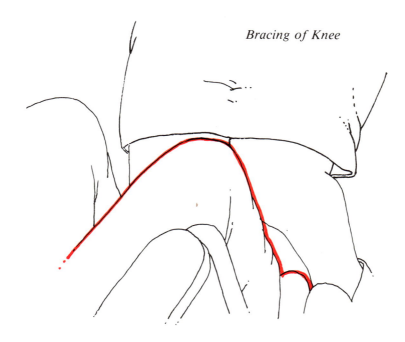

Bracing of Knee

Chair to Wheelchair

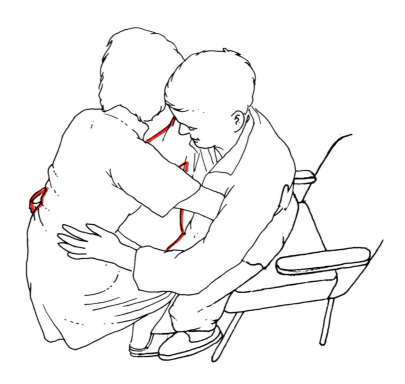

Procedure

- the wheelchair is positioned at right angles to the chair in which the patient is sitting so that he will be transferring towards the **affected side**.
- the brakes of the wheelchair are securely engaged and both footrests and the chair arm on the side of the patient are removed.

Reason

- encourages weight bearing on the **affected leg**.
- increases awareness of the **affected side**.
- ensures the stability of the wheelchair during the transfer.

Procedure

- placing a supporting hand on the **affected scapula**, the operator braces the **affected knee** on either side.

Reasons

- provides the proper support and stability for the patient.
- prevents shoulder joint injury.
- encourages weight bearing through both lower limbs.

Chair to Wheelchair (cont.)

Procedure

- bringing his hips to the edge of the chair and with feet flat on the floor, the patient leans forward to raise his hips off the chair.
- the operator guides the patient's movement assisting as necessary.
- it is only necessary to **stand part ways**.

Reasons

- ensures equal weight bearing through both feet.
- standing part ways requires less assistance from the operator than erect standing.

Procedure

- the patient is pivotted to the wheelchair.
- the patient leans forward and bends both knees when sitting guided by the operator.

Reasons

- encourages the participation of the patient independently with support from the nurse.

Note

- the above procedure is easily performed by one operator.
- with two people, the second operator is positioned between both the chair and wheelchair on the **affected side** of the patient and will guide the hips of the patient.
- the brakes **must** be firmly in place before the transfer commences.

48

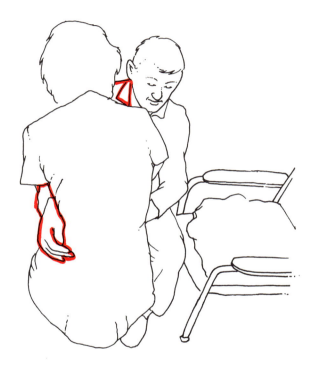

Transfers (cont.)

Wheelchair to Toilet

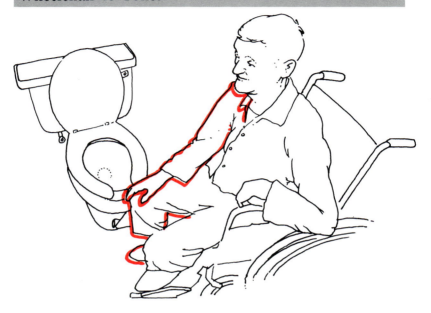

Procedure

- the wheelchair is positioned so that the patient will be transferring **towards the affected side**.

Reasons

- increases the awareness of the **affected side** and further encourages symmetrical use of the lower limbs.

Note

- ensure the brakes of the wheelchair are engaged and footrests are removed or out of the way.

Procedures

- a supporting hand is placed on the **affected scapula** of the patient.
- the **affected knee** is braced on either side by the knees of the operator.

Reasons

- provides support and stability for the patient where it is required most.

Note • offer assistance only when necessary.

Procedure

- the patient brings both hips to the front of the chair.
- the patient leans forward to raise the hips off the chair.
- it is only necessary to **stand part ways**.

Reasons

- ensures equal weight bearing through both feet.
- erect standing requires more assistance from the operator than standing part ways.

Procedure

- pivot the patient to the toilet seat which is at an angle of ninety degrees to the wheelchair.
- the patient bends both knees to sit.

Reasons

- pivoting is easily performed with minimal energy expenditure.
- encourages the active participation of the patient.

Note

- early use of the toilet rather than a bedpan is often preferred by most patients.

Toilet to Wheelchair

The procedure and reasons for transferring from the toilet back to the wheelchair are reversed but identical to the chair to toilet transfer.

In most washrooms, there may not be enough space to transfer both from the chair to the toilet and back to the chair through the **affected side** of the patient. In such instances convenience should prevail.

Transfers (cont.)

From Chair or Wheelchair to Standing (Assisted by two operators)

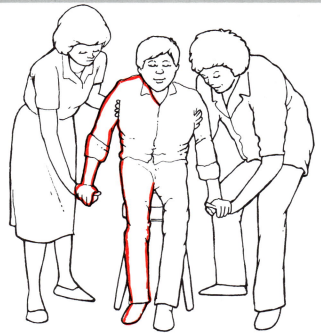

Procedure

- the operators stand on either side of the patient.
- when a wheelchair is being used the brakes must be securely engaged and the footrests moved out of the way.
- each operator places one supporting hand into the axillae of the patient.
- the other supporting hand is placed securely into the hand of the patient.
- the patient is encouraged to lean on the hands of the operators.

Reasons

- provides the patient with maximal support.
- prevents any damage to the shoulder joint.

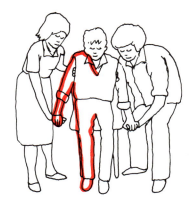

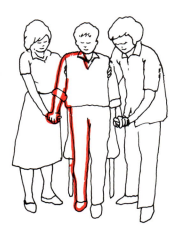

Procedure

- the patient brings his hips to the front of the chair.
- the patient's feet are flat on the floor with the **affected**
- **foot** slightly further back than the sound foot.
- the patient leans into the hands of the operators and moves forward and upward into the standing position
- straightening both legs.

  the operators assist as is necessary.

Reasons

- encourages equal and symmetrical weight bearing through both of the patient's upper limbs.
- allows the patient to experience the sensation of standing up in a normal manner.

Note

- when the patient is more independent, a single operator would support the patient on the **affected side.**
- when the patient sits down again the same procedure is followed but in reverse order.

From Chair or Wheelchair to Standing
(Assisted by one operator)

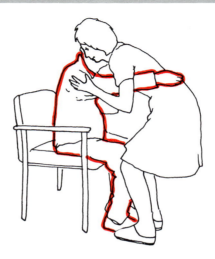

Procedure

- the operator is positioned in front of the patient, a supporting hand is placed on the **affected scapula** of the patient, the **affected knee** of the patient is braced on either side with the knees of the operator.
- when transferring from a wheelchair ensure that the brakes are securely engaged and the footrests are removed or out of the way.

Reasons

- in addition to encouraging normal weight bearing on the **affected limb**, this procedure provides maximum safety for the patient and reduces the likelihood of injury to the operator.

Note

- provide assistance only when necessary.

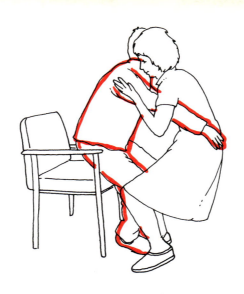

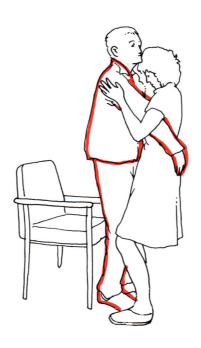

From Chair or Wheelchair to Standing (Independently by the patient)

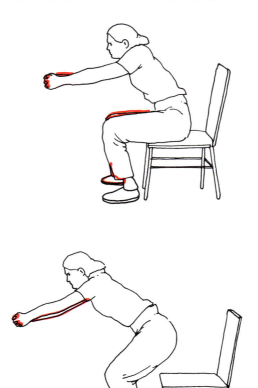

Procedure

- where a wheelchair is being used the brakes must be engaged and the footrests swung away or removed.
- the patient clasps both hands together and reaches forward with the arms.
- the patient leans forward, raising both hips off the chair.
- the knees move forward so that the weight of the patient is over the feet.
- the patient straightens both knees and stands upright taking **equal** weight on both legs.

Reasons

- prevents the appearance of non-functional patterns of spasticity.
- promotes equal weight bearing through both feet.
- encourages the use of the **affected side** of the patient.
- promotes symmetrical movement of the limbs.
- encourages normal movement.

Note

- the nurse may assist in necessary.
- this somewhat advanced procedure may not be attainable in some patients, however it should be encouraged if possible.
- when the patient sits down again the same procedure is followed but in reverse order.

Position and Support of the Operators

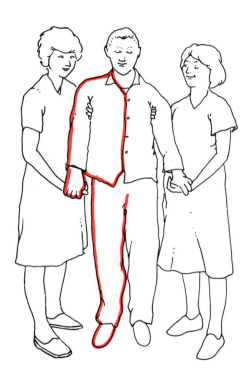

Procedure

- the operators stand on either side of the patient.
- one supporting hand is placed well into the axilla of the patient.
- the other supporting hand holds the hand of the patient.
- the patient is encouraged to lean on the hand of the operator.

Reasons

- provides maximal support to the patient.
- encourages equal weight bearing through both feet.
- prevents damage to the shoulder joint.
- encourages equal and symmetrical weight bearing through the upper limbs of the patient.

Note

- when the patient is more independent, a single operator would support the patient on the **affected side** only.
- the patient may be able to begin walking from this position.

Correct Hand Hold When Standing

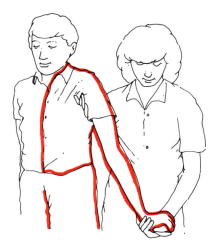

- the palm of the operator's hand faces upwards and the palm of the patient faces downwards.
- the patient **leans** through the **heel** of his hand.

59

Walking the Patient

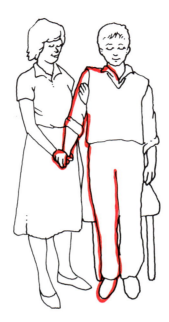

Procedure

- ensure the patient has correct standing posture particularly, the head in the midline position, the eyes facing forward, and equal weight bearing through the feet.

Reasons

- promotes symmetrical body alignment and ensures **normal** sensory stimulation.

Procedure

- the patient shifts weight on to the **affected leg** and takes a short step forward with the non involved leg.
- the operator encourages the patient to bear weight on the **affected leg** when the sound leg is swinging forward. Initially this will be difficult and some assistance may be required.
- when swinging the **affected leg** forward the patient should be encouraged to make a step of equal length and strike the floor with the heel in the normal manner.

Reasons

- weight transfer allows the opposite foot to be brought forward with less effort on the part of the patient.
- promotes symmetrical movement of the limbs.
- encourages the use of the **affected side**.
- allows relearning of a normal gait pattern throughout the rehabilitation process.
- prevents the acquisition of an abnormal gait pattern.

Note

- provide assistance as necessary to ensure as near normal a gait as possible.
- this is an advanced procedure and is a progression from the two operator method.

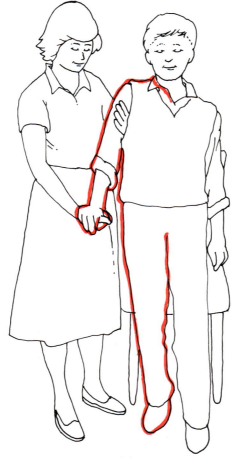

Range of Motion Exercises

General Guidelines

1. Approach the patient from the **affected side**.
2. Encourage the patient to actively participate as soon as possible.
3. Ensure that all body parts which are not being moved are resting in the appropriate supported positions.
4. Upon completion of the task, the limb must be returned to the original proper resting position.

Important:

1. Do not move the limb through ranges of movement which cause the patient pain.
2. Avoid any movement which results in an increase in spasticity.

UPPER LIMB

Procedure

1) • in sitting or lying, the patient clasps both hands together interlacing fingers (see Figure 1).
  reaching forward, the arms are raised above the head and lowered slowly.
  the elbows can also be flexed and extended while reaching forwards.
2) • sitting at a table, the patient clasps both hands together.
  the hands are brought to the mouth and then lowered slowly by flexing the elbow joints (see Figure 2).
3) • sitting at a table with both hands clasped together.
  the patient **slowly** moves the hands to the right then left with movement taking place at the wrist joint.
  slowly lift just the hands off the table and lower again (see Figure 3).

Reasons

- promotes symmetrical movement of the limbs.
- provides independent exercises beneficial to the patient.
- maintains range of movement of upper limb.
- encourages active movement of **affected limb**.
- reduces the likelihood of the onset of painful shoulder which will compromise rehabilitation.
- encourages the patient to touch the **affected hand** thus enhancing sensory appreciation.

1)

2)

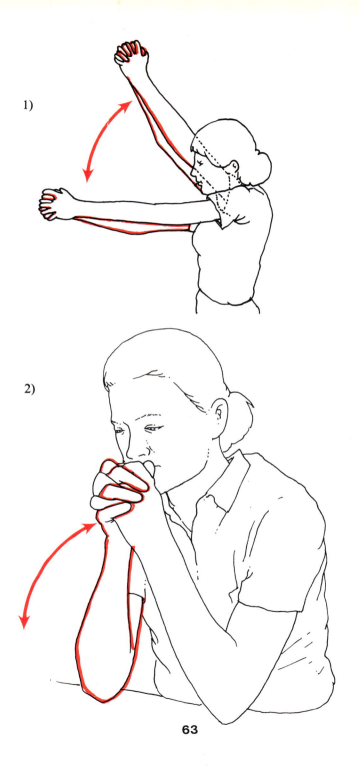

3)

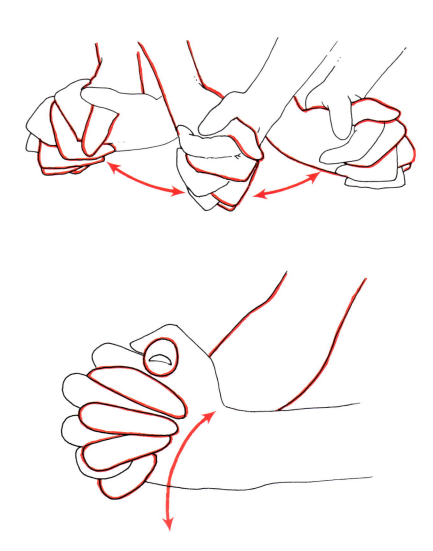

Note

- the patient should only assist with the sound limb as much as is necessary to complete the movement smoothly and without increasing spasticity.
- each exercise should be done several times daily (a few repetitions often).

Important:

Do NOT take the patient's shoulder joint into elevation through abduction in lying as this will damage the shoulder joint causing marked pain and discomfort.

The use of triangular bandage slings are NOT recommended. They support the limb in a non-functional position and encourage disuse of the **affected arm**. In addition this type of sling is ineffective in relieving shoulder subluxation. If support, in addition to careful positioning using pillows and tables, is thought to be necessary for the affected shoulder joint, address the concern to the attending physiotherapist.

Range of Motion Exercises (cont.)

LOWER LIMB

4)

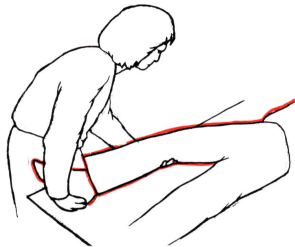

Procedure

- support the **affected limb** at the heel and under the knee joint (Figure 4).

5)

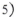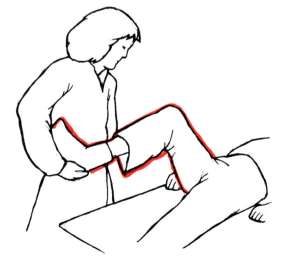

Procedure

- assist the patient to bring his knee toward his chest and to slowly straighten the knee out again (Figure 5).

Reason

- helps maintain range of movement at the knee and hip joints.
- encourages the patient to independently attempt to move the **affected limb**.
- encourages the sensation of normal movement.

Procedure

- the patient bends up both knees and raises the hips off the bed pressing both feet into the bed (bedpan procedure).
- the patient lowers his hips slowly.

Reasons

- prevents loss of hip extension.
- encourages weight transfer through the **affected leg**.

Note

- the patient should be encouraged to participate as much as possible.
- sometimes it is necessary to stabilize the feet of the patient.

Activities of Daily Living (A.D.L.)

General Guidelines

1. Encourage the patient to be as independent as possible.
2. Approach the patient from his **affected side**.
3. Encourage symmetrical lying or sitting position.
4. When task is one-handed, the **affected arm** must be supported and placed in the patient's field of vision.
5. Involvement of the **affected limb** in A.D.L. tasks should be encouraged in an auto assisted manner where appropriate.

Note

- the occupational therapist can offer further guidance and instruction in A.D.L.

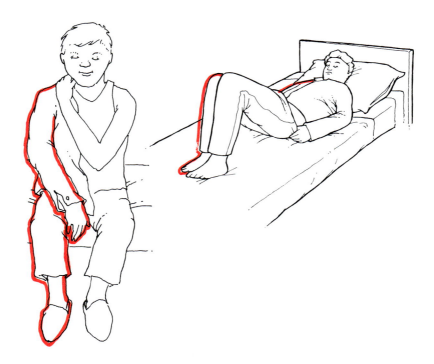

- dressing. Shirt: dress the **affected limb** first.
  Trousers: once the trousers have been placed over the feet the bridging procedure described previously (page 24) can be used to complete the task.

- hair grooming

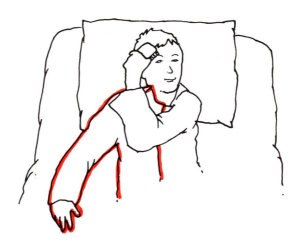

- shaving

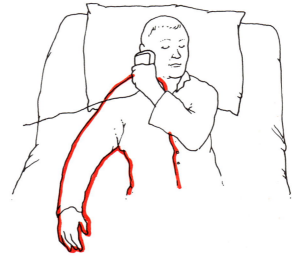

- face washing

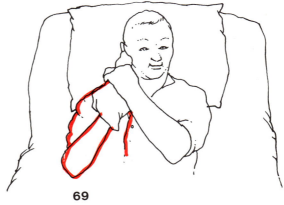

Conclusion

This publication is designed to present current rehabilitation concepts used in the management of the acute stroke patient.

A consistent team approach in the early stages will ensure tht the maximum functional potential of the patient will eventually be achieved.

Current rehabilitation efforts focus on the re-education of the affected side while at the same time preventing complications and suppressing spasticity.

By coordinating their efforts nursing and physiotherapy will complement the role of each other and ensure that the patient has the opportunity to reach his maximum physical potential.

Selected Glossary

Abnormal Muscle Tone: Deviation from the normal state of muscle tone and characterised by flaccidity or spasticity in specific muscle groups.

Abnormal Patterns of Spasticity: Increases in tone of specific muscle groups consistent with lower level uninhibited reflex activity.

Abnormal Primitive Reflexes: Abnormal patterns of spasticity. Present in the newborn but is modified with CNS maturation allowing sophisticated movement. Patterns reappear following damage to CNS.

Activities of Daily Living: Functional activities associated with care of the person (for example: bathing, grooming and eating).

Acute care: The period immediately following the occurence of the stroke and extending until the person leaves the acute hospital setting.

Affected Side: The side of the body demonstrating symptoms. Contralateral to the involved cerebral hemisphere.

Balance mechanisms: Automatic and discrete muscle activity responsible for maintaining postural equilibrium.

Body Image: The appropriate awareness and appreciation of the position of body segments and their relationship to each other.

Bridging: Procedure in which the patient, lying on his back with hips and knees in flexion, raises the hips up by pressing the feet into the bed.

Long Sitting: The patient is sitting up in bed with the knee joints in extension.

Neglect: Inability of the patient to attend to or use the affected side of the body. Often a result of parietal lobe disturbance but may also be an acquired response as a result of disuse.

Range of Motion Exercises: Movements carried out in an effort to maintain full range of movement at joints which cannot be moved in the normal independent manner by the patient. They may be performed by a second person (passive), by the patient himself (auto-assisted) or by a second person with a contribution from the patient (active-assisted).

Re-education: Treatment specifically designed to enable the patient to reacquire a functional competency.

Rehabilitation: The process undertaken by the patient to enable the reaching of full functional potential.

Sensation: Sensory input from exteroceptors and proprioceptors. Normal sensory appreciation is an essential ingredient of normal movement.

Sound Side: The side of the body with normal or near normal function. Ipsilateral to the involved cerebral hemisphere.

Supine: The patient is lying totally on his back.

Symmetry: The situation where both halves of the body contribute to the achievement of functional activity by working together in a highly coordinated manner.

Suggested Further Reading

BOBATH, B: *Adult Hemiplegia: Evaluation and Treatment.* William Heinemann, London, 1978.

JOHNSTON, K and OLSON, E: *Application of Bobath Principles for Nursing Care of the Hemiplegic Patient.* A R N, March–April, 1980 (8–11).

JOHNSTONE, M: *Restoration of Motor Function in the Stroke Patient.* Churchill Livingstone, Edinburgh, 1978.

PARRY, A and EALES, C: *Handling the Early Stroke Patient at Home and in the Ward.* Nursing Times, October 28, 1976, (1680–1683).

PARRY, A and EALES, C: *The Ambulant Stroke Patient at Home and in the Ward.* Nursing Times, November 4, 1976 (1726–1730).

PARRY, A and EALES, C: *The Geriatric Stroke Patient at Home and in the Ward.* Nursing Times, November 11, 1976 (1763–1765).

TODD, J: *Physiotherapy in the Early Stages of Hemiplegia.* Physiotherapy, 60, 336–342 (1974).

Acknowledgements

The Nova Scotia Heart Foundation who funded the development and evaluation of this book.

Derek Sarty for his outstanding contribution to the production of this publication.

Bruce Moxley and The Division of Instructional Resources, Faculty of Dentistry, Dalhousie University for their advice, encouragement and flexibility.

The patients and staff of the Victoria General Hospital, Halifax, Nova Scotia for their invaluable support and cooperation.

The faculty and staff of the School of Physiotherapy, Dalhousie University for their encouragement and enthusiasm.

Dr. C.W. McCormick, Division of Neurology, Faculty of Medicine, Dalhousie University, for his support.